THE SIMPLE LIFE - LIFE BALANCE REBOOT

The Three-Legged Stool for Health, Wealth and Purpose

GARY COLLINS, MS

THE
SIMPLE
LIFE

The Simple Life Series (An Introduction to The Simple Life)

The Simple Life - Life Balance Reboot: The Three-Legged Stool for Health, Wealth and Purpose

(First Edition)

Printed in the United States of America

Copyright ©2020

Published by Second Nature Publishing, Albuquerque, NM 87109

For information about special discounts for bulk purchasing, and/or direct inquiries about copyright, permission, reproduction and publishing inquiries, please contact Book Publishing Company at 888-260-8458.

DISCLAIMER OF WARRANTY

TABLE OF CONTENTS

Get Your Free Goodies!   5
Other Books by Gary Collins   7

1. Part 1 - Why is Life Balance So Hard?   9
2. Part 2 - Leg #1: Optimal Health - The Foundation   21
   of Life Balance
3. Part 3 - Leg #2: Being Debt Free - Why Money   34
   Equals Freedom
4. Part 4 - Leg #3: Life Purpose - Finding Your Road   45
   Map to Happiness

Final Thoughts - Tying it All Together   55
Did You Enjoy This Book? You Can Make A Big   57
Difference and Spread the Word!
About Gary Collins   59
Other Books by Gary Collins   61
Notes   63

GET YOUR FREE GOODIES!

Get Your Free Goodies and Be a Part of My Special Community!

Building a solid relationship with my readers is incredibly important to me. It's one of the rewards of being a writer. From time to time, I send out an email to what I call "The Simple Life Insider's Circle" (never spammy, I promise) to keep you up to date with special offers and information about anything new I may be doing. I've moved away from using social media in the pursuit of a simpler life, but I'd love to stay connected with you via my Insider's Circle.

If that's not enough enticement, when you sign up, I'll send you some spectacular free stuff!

1. **The Five Simple Life Success Principles.**
2. **A free chapter from *The Simple Life Guide To Decluttering Your Life*, where I discuss topics most decluttering books are afraid to talk about.**
3. **A free chapter from *The Simple Life Guide To***

Financial Freedom on why your house is probably making you broke.

4. A free chapter from *The Simple Life Guide To Optimal Health* about the dirty little secrets of the supplement industry, and tips on how to make informed purchase decisions.
5. 10% off and free shipping on your first order at The Simple Life website.

You can get these goodies by signing up for my mailing list at:

http://www.thesimplelifenow.com/startsimple

OTHER BOOKS BY GARY COLLINS

The Simple Life Guide To Financial Freedom: Free Yourself from the Chains of Debt and Find Financial Peace

The Simple Life Guide To Decluttering Your Life: The How-To Book of Doing More with Less and Focusing on the Things That Matter

The Simple Life Guide To RV Living: The Road to Freedom and the Mobile Lifestyle Revolution

The Simple Life Guide To Optimal Health: How to Get Healthy and Feel Better Than Ever

The Beginners Guide To Living Off The Grid: The DIY Workbook for Living the Life You Want

Living Off The Grid: What to Expect While Living the Life of Ultimate Freedom and Tranquility

Going Off The Grid: The How-To Book of Simple Living and Happiness

1

PART 1 - WHY IS LIFE BALANCE SO HARD?

You want to be healthier, happier, and more financially independent. But is it really possible to be all three at once?

Doesn't it seem like every time you work hard on getting your financial life together, you end up tired, stressed out, and neglecting your health or even your relationships? Does it feel like every time you manage to eat healthy and workout for a few days, you end up blowing all your progress in a single weekend? And how often do you lay awake at night, staring at the ceiling, frustrated, or disappointed that you're not really living your dreams or even fulfilling your potential?

If you're like most of my readers, this all sounds way too familiar. And I bet you've read a lot of self-help books, tried a lot of systems, and rededicated yourself dozens of times. Yet, years later, here you are. Still not as healthy as you could be. Still not as happy. Still worried about money. Still stressed about how out of balance your life is.

So what's the real issue holding you back? Self-help authors will usually blame motivation. They'll say...

"Most people know what they need to do. They're just not doing it."

If you're sick of hearing this bullshit, I don't blame you. Because that's exactly what it is. Bullshit. If you knew what to do, you'd probably already be healthy, happy, and financially independent, wouldn't you? But you don't know. And that's why I'm glad you took the first step by purchasing this little book, or someone put it into your hands today.

What you're reading is the "appetizer" for a series of books and products that I call "The Simple Life." The Simple Life isn't about becoming a minimalist. It's not about living off the land in a cabin on Walden Pond. It's not even about simplifying your goals or your daily routines. You've probably already heard enough of those platitudes to make you puke.

The Simple Life's mission is to motivate, educate and inspire people to be the best version of themselves in order to find happiness, personal freedom, and purpose in life while helping others, and to give back along the way. Most importantly, it does this in a way that helps you balance your own life. If you want to be healthier, happier, and financially independent, all at the same time, you need to shut the door, close your internet browser, turn off your cell phone, and get ready to read this book from start to finish.

First, let's talk about why all those other self-help books haven't delivered for you…

THE DARK SIDE OF THE SELF-HELP INDUSTRY

Did you know that during the California Gold Rush, phony medicine men made more money selling fake medical cures off the backs of wagons than most people made mining gold?

I know that's a weird way to start the conversation. But I bet you didn't know that's where the term "snake oil salesman" came from, did you? And can you guess where these snake-oil-peddling "False Prophets" are pushing their products today?

Yep. The personal growth world.

That's why, before we get to the meat of this book, I want to tell you what this book is NOT about. It's not about telling you what SOUNDS right, or even what you want to hear.

During the Gold Rush, millions of people came from around the world to California to get rich mining gold. But the False Prophets of that day didn't want to work that hard. And they didn't have to. They knew something that today's self-help authors learned a long time ago…

If you can't get healthy, happy, or rich by hard, honest work, you can do it by promising to teach other people the secrets to health, happiness, and prosperity.

I can prove this too. Next time you're about to buy a self-help book, look into the author's background. I mean REALLY investigate them. The same way you would if they had asked to marry your daughter. While you're looking into the real experience of an author, ask yourself….

"Who is this person, and why should I listen to them?"

Do this with a couple of self-help books over the next 24 to 48 hours, and you'll see *exactly* what I'm talking about. The self-help world is slithering with swarms of silver-tongued False Prophets and snake oil salesmen. I know this because I've investigated these "experts" myself. And I'm no small-time sleuth either.

My BS-finding career began in my early twenties. I started by getting my bachelor's degree in Criminal Justice. Followed by a master's degree in Forensic Science. Then, I worked as a Special Agent for The U.S. Department of State - Diplomatic Security Service, The U.S. Department of Health and Human Services, and for the U.S. Food and Drug Administration.

So, as you can guess, I've spent thousands of hours, over the decades of my career, investigating some of the slipperiest, slimiest criminals and con artists in the United States. I can tell you with 100 percent confidence that ALL of them have a few scary character traits in common. The most important one being that they're masters of making themselves look smarter and more sincere than they really are.

I'll say that again. REALLY let this sink in as you read it...

The most common character trait of high-profile criminals and con artists is that they're masters of making themselves look smarter and more sincere than they really are.

So, when I became an author, by accident, (I explain how that happened in my other books) I decided to size up my competitors. I investigated hundreds of them, and I've been astonished at the devilish deception of some of these authors. Notably, some of the popular ones. I'll share a few details in a minute. But first, I want to answer the question I encouraged you to ask about other authors...

"Who am I, and why should you listen to me?"

WHO ARE YOU GARY AND WHY SHOULD I LISTEN TO YOU?

If you've read any of my Simple Life books, you know that I never ask anyone to do anything I haven't already done successfully myself. Case in point, I'm best known for "Off-The-Grid" books, where I teach people to escape the horror and gridlock of the typical Clutter Clinging modern lifestyle so they can simplify and "happify" their lives. For me, going off-the-grid is more than just moving to a peaceful location.

It's about escaping the ideological "Grid" that's enslaved people like you and I to lives of debt, distraction, bad health, and unfulfilling careers. To this day, my book *Going Off The Grid* is a bestseller... the irony? It was a book that was never meant to be written.

In all my books, I share the detailed (and at times, embarrassing) story of my mistakes, lessons I've learned, and the victories I've enjoyed during my journey out of The Grid and into The Simple Life. The MOST important lesson is that most of the people giving advice about health, money, happiness, and purpose are the same people who keep the machinery of The Grid running.

These "Gridmasters" come in all shapes, sizes, and education levels. They're lurking behind those expensive cherrywood desks in the financial world. They're huddled behind laptops marketing "lose 30 pounds in 30 days without doing anything" diet plans. They're selling tickets to $5,000 motivational seminars. They're selling books on Amazon and in brick-and-mortar bookstores all over the country. They're even embedded in powerful political positions in our government bureaucracies. The Gridmasters are everywhere.

And yes, their books make it into every bookstore you browse online or walk into. Now, don't get me wrong. I've read some terrific self-help books. But the good books, written by honest, knowledgeable Torchbearers have become disturbingly rare since the internet exploded. Maybe you're slowly realizing this. Perhaps you've read dozens of these self-help books, and years later, you're still stuck.

Again, that's why I want to tell you what this book is NOT about. In fact, I'll reveal one more dirty little secret...

REPACKAGED JUNK IS STILL JUNK

Most Gridmasters in the self-help world don't even write about their own ideas. Instead, they repackage stuff written by other authors. I know. They *try* to rip me off all the time. The problem is, they don't fully understand my ideas because they don't practice what they preach. But if you've always secretly suspected this to be the case, here's a disturbing confirmation…

One of my friends has been a ghostwriter and editor since 2009. He frequently turns down projects for clients who want to become a self-help expert by repackaging shit from other self-help authors. So, if you think these people are rare, you're wrong.

Hell, even their personal claims to fame are either phony or ridiculous. Haven't you noticed how a lot of self-help authors started out as the salesperson of some rubber turd infomercial product? And of course, they were the most amazing door-to-door salesperson ever to promote that product! They become rich, got happily married (maybe), and then they decided to "give something back" by writing a book about how they did it all.

Other authors claim to have been in some life-altering car-accident, or maybe they had their "awakening" when their parents stopped paying for college (heard that one a few times). Others simply went into a deep depression after losing their job or being dumped by their girlfriend. After this "crisis," they had some "one night while I was sitting on the beach watching the sunset" spiritual awakening and…PRESTO!

Instant self-help expert!

Imagine how vigorously you shop for a doctor, or an auto-mechanic, or a dentist or a home repair person. Why not be just as anal about the self-help authors you listen to? If you do this, you WILL find that most self-help authors have two things in common.

First, their stories have ZERO to do with becoming an expert on how to help someone else find health, happiness, and prosperity. Second, their "struggles" are usually no different than things you've already experienced and overcome in your own life.

I mean, who hasn't lost a job, or been broken up with, or suffered a serious injury? If these are all it takes to make you an expert, I guess we're ALL experts! But if you're sick of this nonsense and if you're ready for a dose of honest, common sense, this book is for you.

JUST ASK YOURSELF THESE QUESTIONS...

"Why should these people be telling me how to overcome life's most difficult obstacles?"

"Why should they be advising me on how to do things they've never done themselves? And WHY should they be getting paid to do it?"

Smells like snake oil to me.

Bottom line, in my experience, about 99 percent of self-help books are completely useless. But, you and I are going to put a stop to this nonsense. I do my part by providing information about what really works and what doesn't work at all. You can do your part by rigorously investigating EVERY author you read from now on. Myself included.

Debunking all the dogma-laced self-help systems out there takes a lot of effort. It's harder than it sounds. False Prophets are typically great at making it SOUND like they know what they're talking about. Remember what I told you earlier about criminals and con artists: they're masters at making themselves look smarter and more sincere than they really are. It is not about helping you; it is about manipulating you!

So, now that we've got that out of the way, here are a few things you should know about The Simple Life…

GARY'S SIMPLE LIFE PHILOSOPHY

As I mentioned in the beginning of this book, The Simple Life teaches you to make the most of your life by having less, being more, and making a difference in the world. But it starts with being real about the difference between theory and reality. You see, I have a simple philosophy when it comes to teaching and helping people. You start by getting your own shit together. Then, you start helping others. If you think this is just common sense, look at where people go for personal advice these days. Case in point, I'm amazed at how many people try to get healthy by listening to people who are unhealthy.

I call this the "Oprah Winfrey Effect."

Haven't you noticed how millions and millions of people buy Oprah Winfrey's health and diet products? Oprah is a billionaire. She can afford to buy the healthiest foods, hire personal trainers, and go to the best doctors in the world. Still, she continually struggles with her weight and her health. Why in the world would you get your health advice from someone like that?

Sure, Oprah could teach you a lot about starting your own media empire. She did a great job there. But why go to her for health advice? Yes, I know what some of you are saying…

"Gary is fat-shaming Oprah, and everyone who is struggling with their health!"

If you honestly think this way, please return this book for a refund and go buy a romance novel instead. I'm not here to blow sunshine up your ass. Besides, if you want something to get outraged about, I challenge you to investigate the False Prophets in this industry and join me in calling them out. Just a thought.

The second part of my philosophy is just as simple as the first…

If you want to help people by teaching them, you should have what I call a "butt in the seat and time in the salt mines" experience. This is my common sense take on knowledge and experience, as it relates to teaching others. There is nothing wrong with young, ambitious people who want to be motivators. But you have to have real life experience to become an expert. Otherwise, what is your true motivation for helping people?

This is also why I firmly believe no one should write a self-help book while in their 20's. No matter what they have gone through. I went through some pretty devastating times when I was that age. I'm sure you did too. So have most people I know. But at no point back then did I think I had the knowledge and experience to guide people on some of their most critical life choices. Why should someone who hasn't really lived their life be telling you how to live yours?

The third and final part of my philosophy is the simplest of all. Still, it's the one that's hardest for some people to deal with…

I'm a real person. I'm blunt. I swear. I'm sarcastic. I go off on tangents. Sometimes I say things that are outrageous. Most importantly, I tell you what you need to hear. Not what you want to hear. I don't do this to shock people into buying my books either. This is just who I am.

You see, I have a saying when it comes to how I teach The Simple Life philosophy:

"If you are looking to chase butterflies, ride unicorns, and pet bunny rabbits, this is probably NOT the place for you."

So, if you're what I call a "Self-Help Tourist…" or if you have soft, squishy feelings or if you're an "injustice collector" who prowls around looking for things to get offended and to tweet about, you should read another book. But, if you're sick, sick, sick of snake oil and phony self-help theories, you and I will get along. If you're ready to find out how to balance your health, your money, and your life without cramming your life into some stupid self-help system, this book is going to be your new lifeline.

SO, WHAT IS THIS BOOK ABOUT?

Remember what I said in the introduction to this book. False Prophets in the self-help world often say…

"Most people know what they need to do. They're just not doing it."

I'm sick of hearing this bullshit. I know you are too. If motivation was your problem, you'd be in big trouble. My guess is, you're highly motivated, but doing too many of the wrong things. In my opinion, no amount of advice can turn a lazy person into a hard-working person.

Your life is out of balance because you don't know what to do. By the time you're done reading this book, you will know. Again, The Simple Life System teaches you to make the most of your life, by having less, being more, and making a difference. Most importantly, in a way that balances your life. And this book is the cornerstone of The Simple Life philosophy. I call it my "Three-Legged Stool for achieving and living The Simple Life."

During my journey out of The Grid and into the Simple

Life, I've tested and perfected a three-part, common-sense formula for balancing your health, your money, and your purpose/career.

I know it works because I perfected it using decades of **"butt in the seat and time in the salt mines"** experience. It's simple. Imagine a stool with three legs, each one representing these areas of your life…

1. Your Health
2. Your Finances
3. Your Purpose

Imagine what would happen to this stool if you removed any one of these legs. It would fall over, right? Well, that's why your life is out of whack. You can't be financially independent for long without being healthy. Nor can you be healthy and financially independent if you're not living your true purpose. Likewise, with any combination of the above three legs of your life-balance.

If you've tried to work on these one at a time, or two at a time, and not been successful, that's why. If you've tried and failed, to balance all three at once, it's only because you haven't read what's in this book yet. That's about to change. Today!

I say this with confidence because I've used the Three-Legged Stool System to create a simple, prosperous, and happy life for myself. I've also used it for more than ten years to help my clients and readers do the same. I'm confident that if you give it a chance, it will work for you too.

Before we dig in, let me make a confession about what you're going to learn next. There is no "new" information here. Self-help authors often try to fool you with over-hyped promises about "brand new," "cutting edge," or "breakthrough secrets," "life hacks," that will change your life in thirty-days, or less, with little or no effort on your part.

The first thing you'll learn from my books is that their sales tactics are simply an appeal to novelty and curiosity designed to get you to buy more of their stupid books and overpriced products.

I'm not claiming to be some cutting-edge pioneer of a brand-new scientific system. I'm more like a "Torchbearer." I'm here to pass on the common sense and wisdom that has stood the test of time for thousands and thousands of years. A long historical tradition of great men and women have used these principles to advance civilization, fight evil, and to build our society. You've read about them. You've seen documentaries about them.

But behind all their stories is another story. A hidden story. Once that's full of wisdom which we've been buried under heaps of digital age clutter, blogs, e-books, YouTube videos, whitepapers, e-mails, social media posts, and other bullshit noise.

So, if any of the Simple Life Principles sound new to you, it's probably because you've been chasing overhyped promises about "brand new," "cutting edge," or "break-through secrets," which turns out to be nothing more than fluff and nonsense. People like you are getting tired of this crap. They want real answers. And thankfully, a light of timeless, practical wisdom still burns beneath the scrap piles of minutiae. My job is to pass a little of that light on to you.

Let's start with the first and most important leg of The Three-Legged Stool of finding and living The Simple Life...

2

PART 2 - LEG #1: OPTIMAL HEALTH - THE FOUNDATION OF LIFE BALANCE

Maybe you're scratching your head right now and thinking...

"What does my health have to do with balancing my life?"

I'll say with 100 percent confidence: everything!

I've been helping people become healthier and more athletic for decades.

During that time, I've learned that our declining health is the number one reason most people are unhappy or feel unfulfilled today. Life purpose is a close second, which I'll explain as well.

If you doubt this, just ask yourself how many times one of the following excuses has stopped you from doing something...

1. *"I don't have enough energy."*
2. *"I'm too tired to do it now."*
3. *"I'm too tired to think about this."*
4. *"I don't feel good today."*

Or, my favorite one…

"There aren't enough hours in the day."

This is the one most people tell themselves. And it's pure horseshit. The truth is, you're not running out of time. You're running out of energy. And you're running out of energy for one of two reasons…

1. You're trying to cram too much into your schedule.
2. You're unhealthy.

I talk about the first one in my book: *The Simple Life Guide To Decluttering Your Life.* But, in my experience, the second one is far, far more common. The problem is, most of us lie to ourselves about how unhealthy we are. So, before we talk about how to get healthy and increase your energy, let's bust the number one myth about good health…

THERE'S NO SUCH THING AS BEING OVERWEIGHT AND HEALTHY

If this offends you, you're probably in denial about your weight and your health. It might seem mean to suggest you might be overweight, even by ten to twenty pounds. But in my opinion, it's meaner to ignore our country's number one health epidemic simply because someone's feelings might get hurt. It's also my experience that most people are more over-weight than they think.

Being overweight is a health problem. It's also why most people don't have enough energy and have to make up for it by heavy doses of Red Bull and $7 Starbucks lattes with extra espresso shots. If you want proof of how your weight affects your health and energy level, here's an experiment.

First, take an obesity test and find out how many pounds overweight you are. Then, load that much weight into a backpack and wear it from the time you get up to the time you go to bed. So, you're thirty-five pounds overweight; you'll be carrying a thirty-five pound backpack around for the entire day. Or, better yet, find a friend who isn't overweight and have them try this.

See how tired you or your friend are by noon. Then come back and tell me that being overweight isn't messing with your energy level.

Being overweight is a drain on your energy, but that's not all. Carrying extra weight also puts a strain on your joints and muscles. Most people don't know that your body and nervous system process this as stress. The more energy your body wastes dealing with physical stress, the less energy you will have to handle emotional stress. So, being overweight not only messes with your energy level, it makes it harder to stay positive and upbeat.

Being overweight affects many areas of your life, including:

- Energy Level
- Sex Drive
- Memory
- Willpower
- Stamina
- Stress Level
- Confidence
- Sleep Cycles

- Emotional Health
- Vitality
- Joint and Muscle Health
- Finding and Maintaining Healthy Relationships

And finally, if you're overweight, your diet is likely causing you more harm than good. If junk food and overeating is your problem, consider the real cost of unhealthy eating habits. Junk food is expensive and less filling than real food. And if you're eating more food than you should eat, you're blowing a whole lot of money to keep those extra fat cells alive.

So, now we've covered how your health impacts your energy level and your pocketbook. Do you think it impacts your ability to live your life's purpose too? You bet it does.

Are you starting to see why your health is the foundation of living a balanced life? Do you think this could be why you don't have the energy to work harder (and smarter) at achieving your goals? Don't worry. You're not alone in this.

Americans are growing (rounder, not taller) at an alarming rate. After talking to some other health professionals, I asked them if they were witnessing the same thing as I was, and to my surprise, they all said yes. This tells me most people need to rethink what they mean when they say that they're healthy or "in shape."

While writing *The Simple Life Guide To Decluttering Your Life*, I took a few weeks to observe the people around me to see how long it would take to find an obese person. I had no prerequisites (age, gender, race, etc.), other than whether the person appeared to be obese. I did this to prove a point in the chapter dedicated to health, and why it is one of the biggest problems we face while trying to live The Simple Life.

Spoiler alert—it didn't take me very long to find an obese person during this experiment.

Now, in case you're saying...

"Okay, I get it, Gary, but I'm not THAT overweight."

Let's put that theory to the test...

YOU'RE PROBABLY MORE OUT OF SHAPE THAN YOU THINK

The first step to getting healthy is to stop telling yourself that you're healthy when you're not. The second you shed this denial, you'll be ten times more motivated to get truly well.

So, how overweight are you? Ten pounds, or one hundred pounds, the first step is admitting it. This is harder than it sounds because some people have been out of shape so long, they forgot how good their energy level, sex drive, memory, willpower could be if they'd just get in better shape.

I saw a perfect example of weight denial during a recent interview on a podcast. The podcast host had lost well over one hundred pounds. During the interview, he said he didn't realize how big and overweight he was because all of his friends and family looked just like him. At first, I was shocked. Then it sunk in... a great deal of people in our society are obese, but they don't realize it because everyone around them is overweight too. Others have come to accept obesity as normal for them, and some have gone to the extreme of defending obesity as beautiful.

Let's be honest; the human mind is good at adapting. It's our nature. This is why it's so easy to get used to being overweight and unhealthy. Like the podcast host, you can get so used to it that you don't even realize how overweight you are. When you're overweight, it's also hard to imagine how good you *could* feel if you're not living at your optimal body weight.

If you think this sounds mean, imagine how you'd feel if I

were pointing out another life-threatening condition, like cancer or heart disease. What if I was doing it to show people how their choices were killing them? If you think I'm being dramatic, think about this…

The National Institutes of Health tell us that obesity (and being overweight) are the second most common cause of *preventable* death in the United States. In case you're wondering, tobacco-related illnesses were the first.

On top of that, we have marches for cancer, diabetes, and dozens of other deadly illnesses. Yet, we collectively ignore the dangers of being obese or overweight. How compassionate is it to let people die because you're afraid of hurting their feelings? In fact, I'd say that most people are afraid to talk about this because they're so full of themselves or they are scared of the emotional response they might get from having an honest conversation with their loved ones. They care more about what people think of them than they do about helping people by telling them the truth.

So, now that we've nailed the main cause of low energy let's get honest about one more thing.

BEING OVERWEIGHT IS NOT A DISEASE, IT'S A LIFE CHOICE

Getting healthy is your choice. There are plenty of seemingly logical reasons people use to justify their obesity. Do any of these excuses sound familiar?

"I have a bad metabolism."
"I'm big-boned."
"I don't have enough time."
"My insurance doesn't cover…"

When it comes to life excuses to not make positive change, health is definitely at the top of the "it's not my fault" list. Did you know the phrase "it's not your fault," is actually one of the most common (and effective) phrases copywriters use in selling junk food? Another sign of a False Prophet! Again, these people are masters at faking sincerity and manipulating you into believing lies about your own health and wellbeing.

We live in an "it's not your fault" society. We call obesity a disease. We blame it on a "bad metabolism," when, ironically, being overweight is often the cause of a bad metabolism.

But I can't say it any plainer than this: Making poor life choices is not a disease! If it were, being in debt would be a disease. Being in a bad marriage would be a disease. Having a shitty career or a bad driving record would be a disease. And believe me, the Gridmasters and False Prophets would create and market PLENTY of garbage programs, systems, pills, powders, and potions promising to "cure" you of these diseases. But the truth for the majority of people is that your health is the result of your personal choices.

The fact that we consider eating poorly and not getting enough exercise a disease is appalling to me. Would it surprise you to know that humans are the only animals on the planet who do not know what to eat and how to move in order to be healthy? Yet, society has given us a built-in excuse to waddle through life, buy a pair of stretchy pants and blame everyone else for why we don't have the energy to live a balanced and productive life!

Yes, there are some people who are born with, or who acquire, condition(s) which cause them to be overweight or obese. But they're very, very rare. If it's becoming more common today, it's because we're passing down poor genetics (and bad habits) caused by improper diet and lack of exercise. Besides, even if you're not overweight, there are a few simple tests you can do to find out just how out of shape you are. Believe me, most people don't have a clue and are shocked when they see the results. But this is how you start to break the cycle and lay a solid foundation for living a more balanced life. So let's do it…

TAKING ACTION: THE SIMPLE LIFE APPROACH TO GOOD HEALTH

I teach Five Principles in my Simple Life System. I came up with these Principles almost a decade ago, while working with clients on their health. The Five Simple Life Principles are the cornerstone and primary philosophy of everything I teach. They're also the result of decades of trial and error, not only from my own life experience, but from my experience helping others.

Following these Five Principles will keep everything in perspective so you can focus on the things that will truly change your life for the positive. That's why I consider these so crucial in your journey and highly recommend you master them as part of your personal development. I'm going to give you the first two of these Principles now, and if they resonate you, I invite you to get all Five Principles from reading any of my Simple Life Books. And guess what! I offer the Five Principles as a free download when you join The Simple Life Insider's Circle online. For now, let's look at the first two Principles in terms of our health.

PRINCIPLE #1: KNOWLEDGE IS POWER

Earlier in this book, I said that most people don't know how to live a more balanced life. And when it comes to health, there's probably nothing we're more ignorant or in denial about as a society than being overweight. This includes people who assume they're "in pretty good shape." So, when I say "Knowledge is Power," I mean you need to know the truth about how far away you actually are from your goal of being healthy.

Since it's easy to lie to ourselves about this, we'll use three simple tests to see how out of shape you are.

First, look at an online obesity chart and see where you are on it. If you're overweight, don't make excuses about being "big-boned," or that you have a "lot of extra muscle weight," or that you come from a "big family."

Second, look at a "resting heart rate" chart and see how healthy your resting heart rate is. Again, when you get your result, look at it honestly. Don't make excuses. Excuses won't motivate you to take action on your health. Just get your results and move to the third measurement.

Third, look at a respiratory rate chart (that's your average number of breaths per minute), and see how healthy your resting respiratory rate is. Again, don't make excuses if you get a result that makes you uncomfortable or pissed off.

Once you're equipped with honest knowledge about how healthy you are, you're ready to apply the second of the Five Simple Life Principles…

PRINCIPLE #2: AVOID EXTREMES

Okay, so maybe you're panicking about your health now. But, that doesn't mean it's smart to book a gym membership and start hitting the Stairmaster for two hours a day and eating a strict diet of carrots and mineral water. Instead, pick two small habits you can begin today. Pick a "start" habit, and a "stop" habit, like this….

- **Stop** drinking sodas and sugary drinks.
- **Start** walking for 15 – 20 minutes a day.

If this isn't enough, add a third habit: replacing one serving of bad carbs with one serving of vegetables. For example, instead of having that side of fries at lunch, eat some broccoli or asparagus.

That's it. Just start with a few simple habits, and when you're ready, add another habit. Maybe you're reading this and thinking...

"Gary, I just found out I'm in bad shape! Shouldn't I start with more than just a few simple habits?"

Sure, you could. If you want to burn yourself out and quit after two weeks. But here's one thing I've found while helping people get into better health...

SUSTAINABILITY BEATS SPEED

Most likely, you're out of shape because you've normalized the habit of eating a typical Western Diet. This diet is based on two pieces of Gridmaster dogma that are deadly to your health, and your life-balance: speed, and convenience.

Don't worry. Years of research shows that the effects of the typical (unhealthy) Western Diet can, for the most part, be reversed. These studies show that people who abandon the Western Diet for a more natural diet will regain health and reduce their chances of suffering from the usual Western Diet-induced chronic diseases.

To put that in context, if you want a healthier obesity score, resting heart rate, and respiratory rate, start with simple habits that you KNOW you can stick to until they're second nature. But don't try to do it quick and easy, and don't try to pile on too much at once. Remember Principle #2, and that sustainability beats speed every time.

Of course, junk food is made to taste good. The good

news is that you can train your taste buds to love healthy food too. In my experience, most people are overweight because they've been duped by the dogma of speed and convenience.

You can turn this around by eating a more primitive and sustainable diet and by taking your time and building HABITS instead of obsessing over immediate results. If this appeals to you, I invite you to read more about a "primitive diet" in one of my books, *The Simple Life Guide To Optimal Health*. Here are some basics to get you started…

HEALTHY EATING SO SIMPLE, A CAVEMAN CAN DO IT

Imagine what would happen to an obese hunter-gatherer. Modern humans evolved, consuming a diet of natural foods based on actively gathering plant-based foods and hunting animals. Our bodies, though highly adaptive, need specific nutrients that can only be found in nature to function properly. This has been the case for millions of years and for far longer than our modern ways of eating have existed. This nutritional paradigm has only changed in the last few hundred years, thanks to the advent of industrialized agriculture and factory food production.

The prehistoric man/woman concept is an easy tool to use when you become confused about food or health choices. If the modern world as we know it were to end, you and I would have to live off the land like our predecessors. So, what would you eat? What foods would you have access to in your immediate area?

Whenever you have a question about your food selections, just think what a prehistoric man or woman would have had as food choices. Would they have had access to sugary flavored water, processed starchy pasta, high-fructose corn syrup, sugary breakfast cereals and bars, or artificial sweeteners? How about cushy-chaired scooters with shop-ping baskets in the front?

And did the prehistoric man/woman worry about satu-rated fat? Humans before us didn't count calories. They just ate what was in natural abundance around them when they were hungry. They also didn't have gyms with 72 Stairmas-ters lined up in front of 36 Big Screen TV sets with air conditioning blasting them in the face. True, a lot of them died young. But how many died because they were digging their grave with a spoon and fork? More often, they were killed by a predator, or by another human with a spear and a dispute over territory. Others died of non-diet-related illnesses, which we have treatments for today. So don't fool yourself with the myth about their shorter lifespans as having anything to do with their diet.

WHAT YOU CAN DO RIGHT NOW

With that said, I want to give you a list of ten other things you can start doing today. Just keep in mind that sustain-ability beats speed.

1. Identify your health problems and determine what you need to do to change them. For example, are you overweight? Is there pain in your body? Do you have trouble sleeping? Focusing?
2. Schedule at least five hours of physical activity a week
3. Learn how to cook your own healthy food (not donuts)
4. Connect with people with the same healthy mindset and goals as you
5. Identify your motivation (WHY do you want to live longer and have more energy?)

6. List what types of exercise you enjoy
7. Catch yourself if you find yourself blaming others for your health problems
8. Get seven to eight hours of sleep every night
9. Remove unnecessary stressors from your life (see my Decluttering Book if you need help)
10. Stop making excuses and start today!

You may be thinking *"What If I'm Already Healthy?"*

That's great! I applaud your efforts and you're one-third of the way there in terms of living with optimal vitality and simplicity.

SOME FINAL HEALTH ADVICE

Just remember Principle #2 and focus on sustainable habits instead of speedy results. People who overload themselves don't achieve life balance, and they usually quit within a few weeks. Start small, build up some momentum, and some confidence. Make balance the priority. Not speed. Every week or so, recheck your obesity score and your respiratory and heart rates. Keep this up, and don't be in a hurry. The results will come.

Health is the foundation of the Three-Legged Stool, and becoming financially independent comes next...

●

PART 3 - LEG #2: BEING DEBT FREE - WHY MONEY EQUALS FREEDOM

This is the one most people want to start with. But by now, I hope you realize why we started with health. Still, if you're in terrific health, but you don't have the money to pursue your life's purpose, you won't have a balanced life. Instead, you'll have to work your ass off just to survive and keep your bills paid. In time, the financial stress will catch up and make it hard to eat healthy and stay active. This is why your financial life is the second leg of our Three-Legged Stool System.

Before we talk about becoming financially independent, I want to tell you that your health is the first step towards becoming financially independent. I know, sounds crazy, right? But again, think about how your energy level is affecting your ability to get things done at work and at home. Think about how many times you were too tired to sit down and work on your financial goals. This is hard for a lot of people to face. They want to pretend that they can muscle their way through their to-do list by willpower, and that includes their list of financial goals.

Healthy people are more productive and have a higher

earning potential because they can simply outwork unhealthy people. Yeah, I know… a healthy person still needs skills, experience, and specialized knowledge or education. But all other things being equal, a healthy person will outwork an unhealthy person every time. There is no way around this. That's why health is the foundation of becoming financially independent. But there are a few more reasons health is essential for your financial life, starting with this one…

HEALTHY PEOPLE WASTE LESS MONEY

Your physical and financial health can't be looked at as separate things. Not if you want to be honest with yourself. What most people miss is *how* they are related. According to the Joseph Rountree Foundation—the less wealth you have, the more likely you are to suffer from poor health. Likewise, the more wealth you have, the more likely you are to have good health. But don't be fooled into thinking that this means money is the source of health.

A great deal of information in my books is based on my personal experience and career when it comes to advising you on finances and health. For example, to show you how your physical well-being impacts your health and financial well-being, let me share something I explain in detail in *The Simple Life Guide To Financial Freedom.*

On average, it costs about one-third as much money (33.33%) to prepare a home meal equivalent to the meal you eat out. When I first started working with clients on their eating habits, I had them keep track of their food costs. I've used these findings, along with simple national statistics, and basic math to completely debunk the "eating out is an inevitable living expense" objection. Think this sounds overhyped?

Here's an experiment you can try on your own. Go to your favorite drive-through fast food spot. First, log the amount of time it takes you to go from your house to the restaurant and back home again. Then, document the cost of your meal (to include tip if there is any). Finally, add the cost of the gas. Some of you may even want to calculate in a price for your time. For example, if you work for $35/hour, and it took an hour, you may want to add an extra $35 into your findings.

Once you have these numbers, buy the exact same ingredients for a similar meal the next time you go grocery shopping. Keep track of the time it takes to prepare the meal, and the cost of the items. Don't add the grocery shopping time, because you were going to do that anyway.

Which one takes longer and costs more?

I challenge you to REALLY do this and come up with an answer that allows you to keep using lack of time as an excuse to waste money eating out OR to use lack of money as an excuse for not eating healthy.

Good health is the cornerstone of your financial independence, and the clearer you start to see this connection, the more motivated you'll be to get these two legs supporting each other.

Now, moving on from the connection between health and money, let's debunk one of the most significant pieces of financial dogma…

NO MATH = NO MONEY

Here's something the False Prophets won't tell you… If you can't (or won't) learn and apply basic math to your financial life, you'll probably always be broke. I'm sure you've heard the stories about people who win the lottery, or inherit millions, only to blow it all in a few years. Sure, it's easy to say…

"I'd never do that!"

But I bet a lot of those people said the same thing. If you want to test whether this is true, just ask yourself how much basic math you're applying to your financial life. And don't cheat yourself by saying that this isn't necessary. I have never met an individual who is financially independent who lacks basic math skills. I know a lot of people won't want to hear that, which is why most of the False Prophets insist you don't have to be good at math. But this is not true. When it comes to being financially independent, you do not need to be a math whiz. But you do need basic math skills.

Think of math as the ruleset that governs The Grid. Those who understand and apply basic math to their financial life, or to their business and products, prosper at the expense of those who either don't, can't, or won't learn and apply basic math. Banks and financial institutions don't just have more money than us because they're lucky. Instead, they know how to use math to their benefit and to our loss. This doesn't happen because we're dumb or even because we suck at math. It happens because most of us flat out ignore math, while these institutions are busy using it to get rich at our expense.

Think about the rules of a game like tennis, football, baseball, Monopoly, chess, checkers, or even simple card games like Uno, or Go Fish. Have you ever played one of these games against a more experienced person and had them use the "rules" against you? Young kids are masters at this. They invite you to play a game with them. You don't know the game, but you agree to play. So, they explain the rules to you, then halfway through the game, they start using the rules they *didn't* tell you about to beat you.

That's exactly what The Gridmasters and False Prophets do when they use math to set the rules of the financial game. This is also why people who understand the rules of the financial game have a better chance of winning the game. Meanwhile, those who can't, or won't, learn and apply the rules are forced to depend on luck. Think about the last time you played cards with someone who knew how to win. If you won at all, it was probably because of luck.

The same is true of most people in their financial life. They lose because they either don't understand basic math or because they completely ignore it and live by their habits. And we'll talk about these habits, and where they come from, a little later. But no habit can make up for an unwillingness to apply basic math. I'll give you some simple action steps for using math to improve your financial life in a minute. First, let's debunk the deadliest piece of dogma The Gridmasters use to move money out of your pocket and into theirs...

THE MORE YOU OWN, THE MORE YOU OWE

Most people are losing financially because of their attitude about what money is and what it's supposed to be used for. They see money as a means of buying stuff. This is how Americans are ritually initiated into what I call "The Cult of Clutter." In other words, they own too much crap, and that almost always means they owe too much money.

If you're a Clutter Clinger (I know I once was), you know what I'm talking about. The everyday consumer sees money as a means of filling the void of unhappiness with shiny objects. That's why, in my books on decluttering and in my financial book, I focus on changing your attitude about money. Instead of seeing it as a means of accumulating stuff or status, I encourage you to see it as a tool for achieving freedom.

Simply put, money equals freedom—the more money you have, the more potential for freedom you have. The more freedom you have, the less money it takes to maintain that freedom. I dig deeper into this in my financial book. But I want to start thinking about money in a totally different way than you have been taught.

It is no secret most American's are miserable in the daily grind of the average workweek (which the hours keep creeping up) in today's workplace, and the continual hamster wheel of being the ultimate consumer.

For example, let's say you owe $100,000 in student loan debt. Add this on top of all your other expenses, and you'll need to earn more money than your expenses/debt to pay down your student loans. This stops you from going on vacations and from paying off other bills, etc. Every dollar you pay towards servicing your student loan debt is one less dollar you can invest in living the life you want.

Of course, you could move up in your career, make more money, and pay more towards the debt. After some years of hard work, you could pay off this debt.

This would give you access to more of your monthly income. This is as good as getting a sudden raise. So now, because you've eliminated the debt, you have more money to live your ideal lifestyle. This means more freedom to do the things you want to do. And the more monthly expenses you can eliminate, the more *available* money you will have.

Can you see how getting rid of clutter (like debt) is just as good as making more money? The primary difference is that trying to earn more money demands more of your time and energy, again taking away from the life you want to live. Further, if you don't manage your spending well, you'll end up spending the extra money on stuff, and you'll keep accumulating debt. But, if you pay down your debt, you not only have more money, you also have a greater ability to do the things you want without increased time and effort. More importantly, you'll break the habit of spending everything you make AND of accumulating debt.

Why doesn't this happen for most people? Because they're so saddled with debt and other meaningless financial clutter, they're literally too "stuff poor" to live the life they want. Even if they're making a decent amount of money. That's why I say that the drive to have more money can be just as crippling as the drive to collect more crap.

Below are some examples how being a full-fledged member of the Cult of Clutter is making us broke.

- Between 1995 and 2015, consumer debt has skyrocketed. From 2000 to 2017, it doubled to $3.7 trillion, which is in the neighborhood of $11,000 for every person in the United States.
- A GoBankingRates survey in 2016, conducted as three Google Consumer Surveys, each targeted one of four age groups: Millennials, Generation Xers, Baby Boomers and Seniors. They found one in three people had $0 saved for retirement and 23% had less than $10,000 saved for retirement. That's 50% of Americans who have less than $10,000 saved for retirement!
- Another GoBankingRates survey in 2016, found that 69% of Americans have less than $1,000 in savings.
- As of 2020, the United States Government is over $23 trillion in debt—almost four times what it was in 2000. In case you're wondering how this affects you, think inflation, cost of living, etc.
- According to a 2018 article in Forbes Magazine,

Social Security is already paying out more than it takes in and is on pace to run out of money in 16 years.

The above statistics and facts absolutely scare me, and they should scare you too. They're evidence of what life in the Cult of Clutter is really doing to our happiness, freedom, and life balance. And if you think this is fearmongering, just look around at the people you know. How many of them are chained to jobs they'd rather quit because of their pressing financial obligations? How many of them are just two or three paychecks away from financial disaster?

How many of them lie wide-eyed awake at night, indigestion gurgling in their stomach, staring at the ceiling with money worries racing through their minds? What good is it to collect more stuff and more money, when you clutter up your mind with this nonsense?

Here's another thing: Debt also puts time against you. Every year you spend paying down debt is one year less towards saving for your future. One more year worrying, one less year living. This is not to mention the added "time debt" of having to manage and maintain all the unnecessary stuff you've cluttered up your life with. If you want an example of this, just think about how much trouble it is to move all your things from one home to another.

Are you starting to see why your first step towards financial freedom should be to stop buying so much crap and to get out of debt? You can worry about investing and building wealth later. But first, you have to stop the nonsense. Otherwise, you'll just waste any extra money you make or any wealth you build through investing.

I cover more statistics in my *Financial Freedom* book. But I just showed you how poor eating habits, poor math habits, and poor spending/borrowing habits can devastate your ability to become financially independent. If you never take care of these three things, it won't matter how much money you make. So, putting first things first…

TAKING ACTION: The Simple Life Approach to Financial Independence

Let's apply the first two of the Five Simple Life Principles towards your financial life…

PRINCIPLE #1: KNOWLEDGE IS POWER

Never assume that you know how you're doing financially. Instead, look at your monthly expenses compared to your monthly income and to how much debt you have to pay off. Here's an example (for a family of four) of how to comprise a list of your monthly expenses:

1. Mortgage/rent: $1,000
2. Car loan #1: $500
3. Car loan #2: $350
4. Insurance (all house, renter's, auto, medical, etc.): $500
5. Student loans: $700
6. Groceries/eating out: $1,000
7. Clothes: $100
8. Utilities: $200
9. Credit cards: $500
10. Entertainment: $500

Total monthly expenses: $5,350
Total monthly income: $6,000
Leftover monthly income after expenses: $650

Next, figure out how much debt you have and how long it would take for you to pay it off. For example, if you have

$5,000 in debt and can reasonably pay $100 a month (given your current income vs. your expenses as calculated above), you'd divide $5,000 by $100, and get a figure of fifty months.

Divide that by twelve (for a year), and you're looking at more than four years worth of debt. Remember what I said about debt putting time against you? These simple exercises put that into perspective, and it should jolt you out of your denial and light a fire under your ass.

PRINCIPLE #2: AVOID EXTREMES

If you've honestly applied Principle #1, you should be scared about your financial situation. That's good. Just remember that you don't want to burn yourself out trying to do too much too soon. Instead, pick two small habits you can start on today. Pick a "start" habit, and a "stop" habit, like this....

- **Stop** impulse buying (try cash-only spending, no cards).
- **Start** paying a little extra on your smallest debt every month.

If you want to add a third habit, try my easy savings technique. It's simple. Anytime you buy something with cash (which you'll be doing a lot if you use that to stop impulse spending), take the change and put it into a jar. I've been doing this for 30 years and can tell you that those little deposits WILL add up over time. But more importantly, this will get you into the habit of saving money. And that habit will be worth much more in the long run than the money you put in your jar.

Don't be afraid to start small to pay off debt. No matter how depressed you are about how long it will take you to pay off debt, remember that sustainability beats speed and that it's the habit that matters! Here's a checklist I use every time I want to buy something on impulse:

1. Do I NEED to have this?
2. What problem will this solve for me?
3. How will it improve or make my life easier?
4. Do I need it *right now*?
5. Can I afford it?
6. Can I live without it?
7. Will it just sit and take up space?

Again, it's hard to describe the effect that these simple actions will have on your mind and your soul. Once I had accomplished my goal of being debt-free, it was funny how things in my life just kind of got better. I slept better, I had less stress, and I also had a lot more time because I was spending my free time doing things I truly enjoyed instead of working to pay debt.

Most importantly, remember that paying off debt is as good as getting a pay raise. Once your debt is gone, all that money you were paying every month to get out of debt becomes suddenly available. More importantly, you'll already be in the habit of investing it into becoming financially free, instead of spending it on more crap. You'll be ready to start investing it in more important things, like the third and final leg of your life balance stool...

4

PART 4 - LEG #3: LIFE PURPOSE - FINDING YOUR ROAD MAP TO HAPPINESS

The healthier and more financially independent you become, the more "disposable" time, energy, and money you'll have. You'll either use this extra time, energy, and money to make your life and the world better, or you'll find ways to get your life back out of balance. That's why the third leg of our life-balance stool is finding and pursuing your purpose.

I know I personally struggled with filling my time once I decluttered my life and eliminated time-sucking activities. I'm talking about stuff like shopping for shiny objects, which I didn't need, or watching politically divisive news programs. Once you declutter your life, you might be surprised at how many hours a day you waste on unproductive activities like…

1. Social media
2. Watching TV
3. Playing video games
4. Shopping (for unnecessary items)
5. Surfing the internet

6. Smartphone addiction

I'm betting you could easily free up three to four hours a day just by eliminating or cutting back on these six time-wasters. Surprisingly, as I found out myself, it was more difficult than I realized to fill my newly liberated hours with something productive and enjoyable. I think you'll soon find that the best way to do this is to find a meaningful project or hobby to work on, and to use that to hobby discover and eventually pursue your purpose.

This is smarter than trying to launch directly into a quest to find your life's purpose. That's too much pressure if you ask me. As you'll soon realize, discovering and pursuing your purpose is a process, and it takes time to get it right. But, before we get into that, let's talk about why life purpose is more important to your life balance than you think...

LIFE PURPOSE AND LIFE BALANCE

Lack of purpose is, in my experience, the most common cause of the overall unhappiness of people in modern society. People either never think about their life purpose, or they confuse their purpose with their basic roles and responsibilities. For example, some people might say...

"My purpose is to be a good husband and father."

But let's be real here. Every husband is a husband and should try to be a good one. Every father is a father, and, again, they should try to be a good father. It's the same with all the roles and responsibilities in our life. But stating the obvious is not the same as knowing your purpose. Neither is describing the mental or emotional states you enjoy. For example, some people might say...

"My purpose is to be happy."

If you've never made your own happiness a priority, this might be a good place to start. Otherwise, you should be more specific about your purpose. Everyone wants to be happy. So, again, no need to state the obvious.

So what do I mean by *purpose*? I mean putting all the things that are meaningful to you and uplifting to others into a set of specific goals and actions. Preferably, actions that will turn into habits.

Just remember that you don't need to find your purpose right this instant. But, you should start thinking about it as you read through the remainder of this material and as you continue your journey towards a simpler, happier life. I say this because, again, if you don't find something productive and specific to do with your extra time, money, and energy you have, you'll soon be wasting that time, money, and energy on wasteful habits.

And aren't all those time-wasters what created imbalance in your life in the first place? Eating too many junky foods. Buying crap you don't need. Taking on debt. Indulging and reinforcing bad habits. The only lasting defense against this is to find something meaningful to invest your time, energy, and money into. This is why Life Purpose is a crucial leg of your life balance stool. And that's not all…

LIVE BY YOUR PURPOSE, OR LIVE BY YOUR IMPULSES

Having a specific purpose guards us against all the impulsive and self-sabotaging behaviors human beings are so naturally prone to. Think about it; knowing and pursuing your purpose is the only way to create *lasting* happiness. And who blows more money on products they don't need? Happy people, or unhappy people? If you guessed, unhappy people, you're right. And who do you think is more likely to overeat and binge on junk food? Happy people, or unhappy people? Again, if you guessed "unhappy" people, you're right. We don't even need statistics to prove this. It's common sense.

Just think about all the junk you have in your house that you were super-excited about when you first bought it. How much happiness do those things give you now? And how many times do you eat out of boredom or stress? How many cheap or unused items are cluttering up your garage, or your spare bedroom right now? Would you have impulse-bought these things if your everyday life was filled with purpose and happiness? Would you have eaten yourself into poor health? Better yet, would you be more or less likely to tolerate toxic people in your life?

Now, think about this as it related to the first two legs of our Three-Legged Stool: Health, and Money. Finding and pursuing your purpose protects you from indulging in impulsive buying or emotional eating. This is true for all of us. In fact, you probably know at least one person who makes good money working a job they hate, but they waste most of their extra income cluttering up their house with junk.

This is not a coincidence. Unhappy people typically spend more money on "this will make me happy" products, just to make up for the lack of happiness in their life. This is important because I suspect a lot of readers will be afraid to pursue their real purpose for fear of "not making enough money." But does it really make financial sense to hate what you do for forty, fifty, or even sixty plus hours a week, just so you can have the money to buy back *some* of your happiness and end up in debt anyway?

Finding life balance requires that you change your attitude about health and about money. But beyond that, it requires that you change your attitude about how you spend your time and energy. Finding and pursuing your purpose is the smartest way to make this positive change. Especially if you manage to turn your purpose into a vocation. If you love what you do for a living, you'll be in better health, you'll blow less money, and you'll probably live longer and enjoy your relationships more. I say that's more than a fair trade-off. This is why I say that living by your purpose is the best safeguard against living by your impulses.

DISCOVERING YOUR PURPOSE – IT'S SIMPLER THAN IT SOUNDS

I wish I had the magic potion for finding your purpose. I would have stapled a bottle to this book if I did. But I don't, and that's how it's supposed to be because finding your purpose is highly individualistic. There are also many factors to consider like…

- What are you passionate about?
- What's your living situation—married, single, kids, or a caregiver?
- Why are you doing what you're doing?
- Where are you at in your life right now?
- What are your current and future goals?
- What do you most want to give to others?

First, understand that your purpose is rarely static. In fact, for most, it will be a moving target. And very rarely does someone come into this world immediately knowing his or her purpose. So, don't try to define your purpose in anal-retentive detail just yet. Let it happen as you keep asking this question, decluttering your life, and pursuing meaningful hobbies. Remember the Five Principles. Your purpose will reveal itself in time.

Second, I want to emphasize that finding your purpose is done with action—by doing things and by experiencing life and the world. Not just by thinking and planning. Some peoples' purpose is to be the best mother or father they can be. But how will that translate itself into specific actions and habits? For others, like Elon Musk, their purpose being one of the most innovative people in our lifetime. Now that's specific.

Third, remember that your purpose *will* evolve and develop as you do. Like many others, I floundered at first in finding my purpose. I always knew I wanted to help people. That's how I ended up in the military, law enforcement, health, and teaching. But trust me, I'm no life clairvoyant. My purpose has changed and evolved as time has gone by. But it's always been firmly rooted in helping others through my experiences and knowledge. When I first started out as an entrepreneur, two decades ago, I would have been shocked if someone had told me my purpose today would be fulfilled as an author and speaker! So don't be afraid to let your purpose grow as you do.

Fourth, let your purpose have a life of its own. One big lesson I've learned in life is that purpose can't be forced. It has to be found and developed organically. For some, this comes early in life. For others, much later. Your life experiences are going to create and shape your purpose. For example, a friend of mine started out in the stressful world of consulting for technological companies. But he soon found this to be unfulfilling. During this time, he was volunteering and working with underprivileged children on the side. This was where he found his purpose. He left his high-paying job to work for a non-profit helping disadvantaged children, and he never looked back.

Fifth, find a purpose that serves others in some way. In my opinion, modern humans have abandoned the roots of their humanity when it comes to this point. We're all tribal and are nurturing by nature. We've historically relied upon each other for survival. We did this by being a part of small groups (usually less than fifty people), where our primary purpose was using our skills to enhance our survival and ability to thrive in this group or tribe. More importantly, we used these skills to edify the members of our tribe.

Now, think about this. If you were born thousands of years ago, in a hunter-gatherer culture, your purpose may have been to be a hunter and provide food or to be a healer and provide medicine. You also might have had a secondary purpose in the tribe. My point is that you would have *needed* to have a purpose that took your tribe's needs and survival into account.

One thing that was not and would not be tolerated by our nomadic tribal ancestors was selfishness and the hoarding of any sort of resource. This makes the emphasis of the isolated individual, and of consumerism, a very new addition to the mentality of the human species. A pure fabrication of the Gridmasters based on the soul-crushing Dogma of the Cult of Clutter. This should tell you why so many struggle to find their purpose in today's society. It's hard to find your purpose when you're mainly focused on yourself.

Being a realist, I have to admit that simply having a purpose is not going to pay the bills or feed your family. In today's society, we need to have a balance between having purpose and supplying our minimal survival needs. With that being said, I think most people can weave their purpose into their primary source of income. I know this firsthand because I've done it myself and have taught many others to do the same. But it starts with a few simple action steps...

TAKING ACTION: The Simple Life Approach to Your Life's Purpose

Now, let's apply the first two of the Five Simple Life Principles towards your discovering and pursuing your purpose...

PRINCIPLE #1: KNOWLEDGE IS POWER

If you've been living in The Grid your entire life, I don't expect you to know your purpose right away. In fact, it could take you a few years to unravel it, and that's okay. The point is to get started and to avoid any pressure to get this figured out right away. Remember the points we covered in the previous section...

1. Your purpose will probably change a few times
2. Your purpose is better found by action than by thinking
3. Your purpose will evolve as you grow and evolve
4. Your purpose will (and should) have a life of its own
5. Your purpose should serve others in some way

To start finding your purpose, try answering these three questions...

1. What am I interested in?
2. What am I good at?
3. How can the above two help others?

Start with question number one. Give yourself a window of thirty to sixty minutes every day just to look into things that interest you. While it's important to explore your desires without limiting yourself, it's also important not to just randomly look at things online. In fact, try doing all your initial exploring offline in the beginning. Try going to a bookstore. Browse the magazine section, find a few on topics that interest you, and search those magazines for some stories that really grab your attention.

PRINCIPLE #2: AVOID EXTREMES

By now, you know what I'm going to suggest. Pick a "start" habit, and a "stop" habit for finding and pursuing your purpose, like this....

- **Stop** wasting time with things that add clutter or drama to your life.
- **Start** spending a little time every day to work on or learn about something that interests you.

If you have an idea of what your purpose might be, maybe you can add a third habit by looking for ways to turn it into a vocation. But, I can tell you that this step all starts with the question: how can I use my interests and skills to serve other people? If you're good at something and passionate about it, there are likely people out there who will either pay you to do it or to teach them to do it or who will buy a product that you create using your skills. But don't start right out thinking about how you'll make money with your purpose. That would be like trying to build a house by starting with the roof.

But you have to start by asking yourself how your skill can serve others. This is much different than asking, *"how can I use this to make money?"* That's the question the False Prophets in the self-help world probably asked themselves before they decided to write bullshit books and sell them to you, under the guise of "wanting to help." Remember that Purpose is all about happiness, and happiness isn't just about making yourself happy. It's about sharing that happiness with the world and using it to make other people's lives better.

We've already talked about the most crucial action step towards making this discovery happen. Set aside thirty to sixty minutes every day to start exploring your desires and interests. If you can't do this every day, give yourself a three to four-hour window every weekend. But, don't just explore your interests in isolation. Join some groups and connect with other people who are interested in the same things you are. Some of the best ideas and inspirations will come to you during conversations with other people. Connecting with like-minded people will also remind you that your purpose should ultimately be about serving others.

If you do these things, a time will naturally come when you'll be motivated to start acting on what you've discovered. When it does, don't hesitate. Take action. The other two questions above will begin to answer themselves as you do. And the more active you are in living and refining your purpose, the more empowered you'll be to keep the other two legs of your life balance stool strong. The stronger these are, the more time, money, and energy you'll have for pursuing your purpose, and your whole life will become a self-reinforcing habit of personal empowerment. Get started today and see for yourself.

FINAL THOUGHTS - TYING IT ALL TOGETHER

I'll close by reminding you of what the False Prophets usually tell you about creating a balanced and happy life…

"Most people know what they need to do. They're just not doing it."

Again, this is just another load of horseshit. Until now, your life has been out of balance because you *didn't* know what to do. The good news is, now you do. Now it's time to make ALL the areas of your work at once…

1. Your Health
2. Your Finances
3. Your Purpose

Now you know why. Now you know why you've tried, and failed, to balance all three at once. Now it's time to change this. Starting today. But this is just the beginning. Again, this book is the "appetizer" for a series of books and products that I call "The Simple Life." The Simple Life isn't about adding more and more useless "trendy" habits or bullshit that has nothing to do with making your life better and more purposeful. The problem isn't that we don't have enough of something. It is almost always because we have too much of the things the False Prophets have told us we need.

The Simple Life teaches you to make the most of your life, by having less, being more, and making a difference. Most importantly, it does this in a way that balances your life. If you want to be healthier, happier, and financially independent, all at the same time, I invite you to take the next step and sign up and be a part of my exclusive—The Simple Life Insider's Circle. You can do this by visiting my website www.thesimplelifenow.com, and while you are there pick the next book in our journey together. Thanks for reading this book, and welcome to The Simple Life Tribe!

DID YOU ENJOY THIS BOOK? YOU CAN MAKE A BIG DIFFERENCE AND SPREAD THE WORD!

Did You Enjoy This Book? You Can Make A Big Difference and Spread the Word!

Reviews are the most powerful tool I have to bring attention to "The Simple Life." I'm an independently published author. Yes, I do a lot of this work myself. This helps me make sure the information I provide is straight from the heart and from my experiences, without some publishing company dictating what sells. You, the readers, are my muscle and marketing machine.

You're a committed group and a loyal bunch of fans!

I truly love my fans and the passion they have for my writing and products. Simply put, your reviews help bring more fans to my books and attention to what I'm trying to teach.

If you liked this book, or any of my others for that matter, I would be very grateful if you would spend a couple of minutes and leave a review. Doesn't have to be long, just something conveying your thoughts. If you would go to www.amazon.com and leave a review, it would be greatly appreciated.

If you hated this book, and think I suck, I would appreciate an email conveying your thoughts instead of writing a scathing review... that doesn't do either one of us any good.

Thank you!

Gary Collins

ABOUT GARY COLLINS

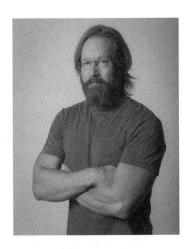

Gary Collins has a compelling background that includes military intelligence, Special Agent for the U.S. State Department Diplomatic Security Service, U.S. Department of Health and Human Services, and U.S. Food and Drug Administration. Gary's expert knowledge brings a much-needed perspective to today's areas of simple living, health, nutrition, entrepreneurship, self-help, and being more self-reliant. He holds an AS degree in Exercise Science, BS in Criminal Justice, and MS in Forensic Science.

Gary was raised in the High Desert at the basin of the Sierra Nevada mountain range in a rural part of California. He now lives off-the-grid part of the year in a remote area of NE Washington State and spends the rest of the year exploring in his travel trailer with his trusty black lab Barney.

Gary considers himself lucky to have grown up in a small town where he enjoyed fishing, hunting, and anything outdoors from a very young age. He has been involved in organized sports, nutrition, and fitness for almost four decades. He is an active follower and teacher of what he calls "life simplification." Gary often says:

"Today, we're bombarded by too much stress, not enough time for personal fulfillment, and failing to take care of our health... there has to be a better way!"

In addition to being a best-selling author, Gary is a highly sought after speaker in numerous areas, as they relate to self-improvement and life simplification. He has taught at the University level, consulted and trained collegiate athletes, and been interviewed for his expertise on various subjects by CBS Sports, Coast to Coast AM, The RT Network, and FOX News, to name a few.

His website www.thesimplelifenow.com, Podcast "Your Better Life," and ***The Simple Life*** book series (his total lifestyle reboot), blows the lid off of conventional life and wellness expectations and is considered essential for every person seeking a simpler, and happier life.

NOTES